Chia Seeds Guide for Beginners

The Importance of Chia Seeds

By

Yestin Wendell

Table of Contents

CHAPTER 1

Introduction

1.1 Understanding Chia Seeds

Chia seeds, scientifically known as Salvia hispanica, are small, nutrient-dense seeds that have gained remarkable popularity in recent years due to their exceptional nutritional content and versatile uses. Originating from Central America, these seeds have a rich history deeply rooted in ancient civilizations like the Aztecs and Mayans, where they were a staple in their diets for centuries.

Chia seeds are incredibly tiny, oval-shaped seeds with a neutral taste, which makes them easy to incorporate into various dishes without significantly altering the flavor. Their neutral profile allows them to complement both sweet and savory dishes, making them a versatile ingredient in modern cuisines.

These seeds are a nutritional powerhouse, packed with essential nutrients. Despite their size, chia seeds are abundant in omega-3 fatty acids, particularly alpha-linolenic acid (ALA), which is crucial for heart health, brain function, and reducing inflammation in the body. Additionally, they boast an impressive array of nutrients including fiber, protein, antioxidants, vitamins (like vitamin B, vitamin E), and minerals (such as calcium, phosphorus, magnesium, and manganese).

One of the unique properties of chia seeds is their ability to absorb liquid and form a gel-like substance when soaked. This characteristic makes them an excellent binding agent in recipes and a popular ingredient in making puddings, jams, or as an egg substitute in vegan baking.

Beyond their nutritional benefits, chia seeds offer various health advantages. They are known for promoting digestive health due to their high fiber content, aiding in proper digestion and preventing constipation. Moreover, their ability to absorb liquid and expand in the stomach may contribute to a feeling of fullness, potentially aiding in weight management by reducing appetite.

Chia seeds have gained attention for their potential role in managing blood sugar levels. Some studies suggest that the gel-forming property of chia seeds may slow down the conversion of carbohydrates into sugar, potentially helping to stabilize blood sugar levels after meals.

Their versatility extends beyond the realm of food; chia seeds are also used in wellness practices. Chia seeds are sometimes incorporated into skincare routines due to their antioxidant properties, which may help combat skin aging and damage caused by free radicals.

Despite their numerous benefits, it's important to consume chia seeds in moderation. Excessive intake might lead to digestive issues for some individuals due to their high fiber content. Additionally, people with certain medical conditions or those taking medications should consult a healthcare professional before incorporating chia seeds into their diet, as they may interact with medications or exacerbate certain health conditions.

chia seeds stand as a nutritional powerhouse deeply embedded in history yet continuing to make waves in modern nutrition and culinary practices due to their exceptional nutritional content, versatile uses, and potential health benefits. Understanding the properties and benefits of chia seeds allows individuals to make informed decisions about incorporating this superfood into their diets for improved overall health and wellness.

1.2 Historical Significance

The historical significance of chia seeds dates back thousands of years, deeply intertwined with the cultural heritage of Central America.

Originating from regions like Mexico and Guatemala, chia seeds were a fundamental part of the diet and culture of ancient civilizations such as the Aztecs and Mayans.

In these ancient societies, chia seeds were revered for their remarkable nutritional properties and were considered a staple food. The Aztecs, in particular, held chia seeds in high regard for their ability to provide sustained energy and endurance, especially for warriors and messengers. In fact, "chia" itself is believed to have derived from the Mayan word for "strength."

These seeds were so valued that they held a significant place in religious ceremonies, trade, and even as offerings to the gods. Chia seeds were used as a form of currency and were often offered in tribute to Aztec rulers.

Beyond their dietary significance, chia seeds had practical uses as well. The gel-like substance formed when the seeds were mixed with water made them a useful ingredient in creating paints, medicines, and even as a means of hydration for long journeys.

However, with the arrival of Spanish conquistadors and the subsequent colonization of the Americas, many indigenous traditions, including the cultivation and consumption of chia seeds, declined. Chia was suppressed and replaced by other crops introduced by the colonizers.

For centuries, chia seeds remained relatively obscure outside of their native regions until their resurgence in recent decades as a "superfood" in modern health and wellness circles. Their nutritional benefits, rich history, and versatility in cooking have led to a renewed global interest in chia seeds, re-establishing their importance in contemporary diets.

The revival of chia seeds not only highlights their nutritional significance but also serves as a testament to the resilience of ancient wisdom and traditional foods, emphasizing the importance of incorporating these time-tested superfoods into today's diverse diets.

CHAPTER 2

Nutritional Profile

2.1 Macronutrients in Chia Seeds

Chia seeds are renowned for their exceptional nutritional content, boasting a well-balanced profile of macronutrients that contribute to their status as a superfood.

Macronutrients in Chia Seeds:

1. Protein:

Chia seeds are a notable plant-based source of protein. They contain all nine essential amino acids, making them a complete protein source, which is rare among plant foods. Protein is essential for muscle repair, growth, and overall cellular function.

2. Fiber:

These tiny seeds are incredibly rich in dietary fiber, with a high content of both soluble and insoluble fiber. The soluble fiber in chia seeds can absorb water, forming a gel-like substance that aids digestion and promotes a feeling of fullness. Insoluble fiber adds bulk to stool and supports regular bowel movements.

3. Healthy Fats:

Chia seeds are particularly renowned for their omega-3 fatty acid content, predominantly alpha-linolenic acid (ALA). Omega-3s play a vital role in heart health, brain function, and reducing inflammation in the body.

Additionally, chia seeds have a favorable omega-3 to omega-6 ratio, which is beneficial for overall health.

4. Carbohydrates:

Despite being a rich source of fiber, chia seeds are relatively low in digestible carbohydrates. The majority of their carbohydrate content comes from fiber, contributing to their low net carbohydrate count, making them a popular choice for those following low-carb diets.

5. Calories:

Considering their small size, chia seeds are calorie-dense. However, the high nutrient density makes them a valuable addition to the diet, offering substantial nutritional benefits for a relatively modest caloric intake.

6. Minerals and Vitamins:

Chia seeds are packed with essential minerals such as calcium, phosphorus, magnesium, manganese, and trace amounts of other minerals like zinc and copper. They also contain various B vitamins, vitamin E, and some vitamin A.

7. **Antioxidants:**

Chia seeds contain antioxidants that help combat oxidative stress and protect cells from damage caused by free radicals. These antioxidants contribute to overall health and may have anti-aging properties.

Understanding the macronutrient composition of chia seeds underscores their nutritional value and versatility in meeting various dietary needs. Incorporating these seeds into one's diet can contribute significantly to overall health and well-being, offering a range of essential nutrients in a small but potent package.

2.2 Micronutrients and Antioxidants

The micronutrient and antioxidant profile of chia seeds contributes significantly to their status as a nutritional powerhouse:

Micronutrients in Chia Seeds:

1. **Calcium:**

Chia seeds are an excellent source of calcium, crucial for bone health, muscle function, and nerve transmission. They contain more calcium by weight than most dairy products.

2. **Phosphorus:**

Essential for bone health and the formation of DNA and cell membranes, phosphorus is abundant in chia seeds, supporting overall body function.

3. Magnesium:

Chia seeds are rich in magnesium, which plays a role in over 300 enzymatic reactions in the body, contributing to energy production, muscle function, and bone health.

4. Manganese:

A trace mineral found in chia seeds, manganese is important for metabolism, bone formation, and antioxidant defenses.

5. Zinc:

Chia seeds contain zinc, an essential mineral involved in immune function, wound healing, and DNA synthesis.

2.3 Antioxidants in Chia Seeds

1. **Polyphenols:**

Chia seeds are a source of various polyphenolic compounds, including flavonoids and phenolic acids, which have antioxidant properties. These compounds help neutralize free radicals, reducing oxidative stress and inflammation.

2. **Quercetin:**

Found in chia seeds, quercetin is a flavonoid known for its anti-inflammatory and antioxidant effects. It may have various health benefits, including supporting heart health and reducing the risk of chronic diseases.

3. **Chlorogenic Acid:**

Another antioxidant present in chia seeds, chlorogenic acid, has been linked to potential benefits such as blood sugar regulation and improved heart health.

4. Caffeic Acid:

Caffeic acid, a phenolic compound found in chia seeds, exhibits antioxidant properties and may contribute to the seeds' overall health benefits.

Importance of Micronutrients and Antioxidants:

Micronutrients and antioxidants in chia seeds play crucial roles in supporting overall health. They contribute to strong bones, efficient metabolism, proper nerve function, and a robust immune system. Antioxidants, in particular, help combat oxidative stress, which is associated with various chronic diseases and aging processes.

Incorporating chia seeds into the diet, individuals can benefit from these micronutrients and antioxidants, which work synergistically to promote health, protect cells from damage, and potentially reduce the risk of chronic conditions.

Understanding the diverse range of micronutrients and antioxidants present in chia seeds underscores their significance as a nutrient-dense food that can contribute to a well-rounded and balanced diet.

CHAPTER 3

Health Benefits of Chia Seeds

3.1 Heart Health and Cholesterol

Chia seeds offer notable health benefits, particularly in promoting heart health and managing cholesterol levels due to their rich nutritional composition.

Heart Health Benefits:

1. Omega-3 Fatty Acids:

Chia seeds are one of the richest plant sources of omega-3 fatty acids, particularly alpha-linolenic acid (ALA). Omega-3s are known for their cardiovascular benefits, including reducing the risk of heart disease by lowering levels of triglycerides, a type of fat in the blood associated with heart problems.

2. Lowering LDL Cholesterol:

Studies suggest that chia seeds may have a positive impact on LDL ("bad") cholesterol levels. The soluble fiber in chia seeds may help reduce LDL cholesterol, potentially decreasing the risk of plaque buildup in arteries and lowering the risk of heart disease.

3. Balancing Omega-3 to Omega-6 Ratio:

Chia seeds contain a favorable ratio of omega-3 to omega-6 fatty acids. Maintaining a balanced ratio between these fatty acids is important for heart health, as an imbalance may contribute to inflammation and heart-related issues.

4. Blood Pressure Regulation:

The magnesium content in chia seeds may play a role in regulating blood pressure. Adequate magnesium intake has been associated with lower blood pressure levels, which is crucial for heart health.

Incorporating Chia Seeds for Heart Health:

1. Chia Seed Gel:

Chia seeds' ability to absorb water and form a gel-like substance can be utilized to create a heart-healthy gel. This gel can be incorporated into smoothies, yogurt, or used as an egg substitute in recipes to add soluble fiber and omega-3s to the diet.

2. Daily Consumption:

Including chia seeds in regular meals—sprinkled on salads, added to oatmeal or cereals, blended into smoothies, or used in baking—can be an easy way to incorporate their heart-healthy benefits into your diet.

While chia seeds offer promising heart health benefits, it's important to remember that they work best as part of a balanced diet and a healthy lifestyle. They shouldn't be relied upon as the sole solution for heart health or cholesterol management. Consulting with a healthcare professional before making significant dietary changes, especially for those with existing medical conditions or taking medications, is always advisable.

chia seeds' high omega-3 content, soluble fiber, and other nutrients contribute to their potential in supporting heart health and managing cholesterol levels, making them a valuable addition to a heart-healthy diet.

3.2 Digestive Health

Chia seeds are celebrated for their significant contribution to digestive health, primarily due to their exceptional fiber content and unique gel-forming properties.

Fiber Content:

1. Soluble and Insoluble Fiber:

Chia seeds are rich in both soluble and insoluble fiber. Soluble fiber forms a gel-like substance when mixed with liquids, aiding digestion by slowing down the absorption of carbohydrates and promoting a feeling of fullness. Insoluble fiber adds bulk to stool, supporting regular bowel movements and preventing constipation.

2. Promotion of Regular Bowel Movements:

The combination of soluble and insoluble fiber in chia seeds supports digestive regularity. The gel-forming ability of chia seeds helps retain water in the stool, making it softer and easier to pass, thereby preventing constipation.

3. Gut Microbiota Support:

Dietary fiber is known to serve as a prebiotic, promoting the growth of beneficial bacteria in the gut. This, in turn, supports a healthy gut microbiome, which is crucial for optimal digestive function and overall health.

Incorporating Chia Seeds for Digestive Health:

1. Hydration:

As chia seeds absorb water and expand, it's important to consume them adequately hydrated. Drinking enough fluids when consuming chia seeds helps the seeds form the desired gel-like consistency, aiding digestion without causing discomfort.

2. Gradual Incorporation:

For individuals new to consuming chia seeds, it's advisable to start with small amounts and gradually increase intake to allow the digestive system to adjust to the increased fiber content.

3. Versatile Uses:

Chia seeds can be easily incorporated into various dishes to boost fiber intake. They can be added to smoothies, yogurt, oatmeal, salads, or used as a thickening agent in soups and sauces.

While chia seeds offer significant digestive health benefits, it's crucial to consume them as part of a well-rounded diet rich in diverse sources of fiber. Overconsumption without adequate hydration might lead to discomfort or digestive issues for some individuals.

chia seeds' high fiber content, with both soluble and insoluble fiber, contributes to improved digestive health by supporting regular bowel movements, promoting a healthy gut microbiota, and aiding in overall digestive function. Incorporating chia seeds into a balanced diet can be an effective way to enhance digestive health.

3.3 Weight Management

Chia seeds have gained attention for their potential role in weight management due to several factors associated with their nutritional composition and unique properties.

Factors Contributing to Weight Management:

1. High Fiber Content:

Chia seeds are exceptionally high in dietary fiber, both soluble and insoluble. This fiber content aids in creating a feeling of fullness, which may help reduce appetite and prevent overeating. The gel-like substance formed by chia seeds when mixed with liquids expands in the stomach, contributing to a sense of satiety.

2. Low Net Carbohydrates:

Despite their high fiber content, chia seeds have relatively low net carbohydrates. Net carbs refer to the digestible carbohydrates in a food item, which are lower in chia seeds due to their fiber content. This characteristic can be beneficial for those following low-carb diets.

3. Protein and Nutrient Density:

Chia seeds are nutrient-dense and contain a moderate amount of protein. Protein plays a crucial role in supporting feelings of fullness and satiety, which may aid in controlling appetite and managing weight.

4. Slow Release of Energy:

The combination of fiber, healthy fats, and protein in chia seeds contributes to a slower release of energy. This steady release of energy may help prevent rapid spikes and crashes in blood sugar levels, supporting stable energy levels throughout the day and potentially reducing cravings for high-calorie foods.

Incorporating Chia Seeds for Weight Management:

1. Portion Control:

Chia seeds are calorie-dense, so mindful portion control is essential when incorporating them into the diet, especially for those watching their calorie intake.

2. Meal and Snack Additions:

Adding chia seeds to meals or snacks can enhance their nutritional value and contribute to a feeling of fullness. They can be sprinkled on salads, mixed into yogurt or oatmeal, blended into smoothies, or used as a topping for various dishes.

3. Hydration:

Consuming chia seeds with sufficient fluids is crucial to allow them to expand and form the gel-like substance in the stomach. This can help avoid potential discomfort and aid in achieving a feeling of fullness.

3.4 Energy and Endurance

Chia seeds are often lauded for their potential to boost energy levels and enhance endurance due to their unique nutritional composition and properties.

Energy-Boosting Properties:

1. Omega-3 Fatty Acids:

Chia seeds are a rich source of omega-3 fatty acids, particularly alpha-linolenic acid (ALA). Omega-

3s play a role in energy production at the cellular level and are linked to improved stamina and endurance.

2. Complex Carbohydrates:

Chia seeds contain a balanced ratio of carbohydrates, including both soluble and insoluble fiber. These complex carbohydrates provide a sustained release of energy, supporting endurance during physical activities.

3. Hydration:

Chia seeds have the remarkable ability to absorb liquid, forming a gel-like substance. This property helps retain hydration during exercise, potentially aiding in maintaining optimal performance and preventing dehydration, which can impact energy levels.

Endurance-Enhancing Properties:

1. Nutrient Density:

Chia seeds are densely packed with nutrients, including protein, fiber, vitamins, and minerals. These nutrients provide essential support for overall body function, aiding in sustained endurance during physical activities.

2. Electrolytes:

Chia seeds contain minerals like potassium, magnesium, and calcium, which are vital electrolytes. Electrolytes play a crucial role in maintaining proper hydration, muscle function, and energy production, supporting endurance during exercise.

3. Slow Energy Release:

The combination of fiber, protein, and healthy fats in chia seeds contributes to a slower release of energy. This steady energy release may help sustain endurance during prolonged physical activities.

Incorporating Chia Seeds for Energy and Endurance:

1. Pre-Exercise Consumption:

Consuming chia seeds before physical activity, mixed with water or incorporated into a pre-workout meal or snack, may help provide a sustained source of energy for endurance activities.

2. Hydration Mix:

Creating a hydration mix by combining chia seeds with water and a bit of natural sweetener or fruit juice can serve as a natural energy drink that helps maintain hydration and provides sustained energy during workouts.

3. Post-Exercise Recovery:

Adding chia seeds to post-workout meals or snacks can contribute to replenishing energy stores and aiding in muscle recovery due to their nutrient density.

CHAPTER 4

Culinary Uses and Incorporation

4.1 Recipes and Cooking Tips

chia seeds are incredibly versatile in the kitchen, offering numerous possibilities for incorporation into various recipes. Here are some culinary uses and cooking tips to make the most of chia seeds:

1. Chia Seed Pudding:

- Combine chia seeds with your choice of liquid (almond milk, coconut milk, or yogurt) and sweetener (honey, maple syrup) to create a pudding-like consistency. Allow it to sit in the fridge overnight for the seeds to absorb the liquid and create a delicious, healthy pudding. Add fruits, nuts, or spices for extra flavor.

2. Smoothie Booster:

- Sprinkle a tablespoon of chia seeds into your favorite smoothie before blending. The seeds will add texture, thickness, and a nutritional boost without altering the flavor significantly.

3. Egg Substitute:

- Mix one tablespoon of ground chia seeds with three tablespoons of water to substitute for one egg in baking recipes. Let it sit for a few minutes until it forms a gel-like consistency. This is an excellent vegan-friendly replacement in recipes that call for eggs.

4. Baking Ingredient:

- Incorporate chia seeds into baked goods like bread, muffins, cookies, and pancakes by adding them directly to the batter. They can add a delightful crunch or texture to your baked treats.

5. Thicken Sauces and Soups:

- Use chia seeds as a natural thickening agent by sprinkling them into sauces, gravies, or soups. They will absorb excess liquid and help create a thicker consistency.

6. Chia Jam:

- Create a healthier version of jam by mixing mashed fruits with chia seeds. Let the mixture sit until the chia seeds absorb the liquid and thicken it naturally, reducing the need for added sugars or pectin.

7. Salad Topping:

- Sprinkle chia seeds on top of salads or grain bowls to add a nutritious crunch and boost the meal's fiber and omega-3 content.

8. Hydration Boost:

- Make a chia seed drink by soaking them in water or juice. The seeds will absorb the liquid and create a hydrating, slightly gelatinous beverage packed with nutrients.

Tips for Using Chia Seeds:

- **Soak Before Consuming:** To fully benefit from their nutritional properties and avoid any discomfort, consider soaking chia seeds before consuming to allow them to expand and form a gel-like consistency.

- **Store Properly:** Keep chia seeds in an airtight container in a cool, dry place to maintain their freshness and prevent them from going rancid.

Experimenting with chia seeds in various recipes allows you to explore their versatility while reaping their nutritional benefits. Whether you're seeking added texture, thickening agents, or a nutritional boost, chia seeds can be a fantastic addition to your culinary repertoire.

4.2 Baking with Chia Seeds

Baking with chia seeds can be a delightful way to incorporate their nutritional benefits into your favorite baked goods. Here are some tips and ideas for using chia seeds in baking:

1. Chia Seed Egg Replacement:

- Create a chia gel by combining one tablespoon of chia seeds with three tablespoons of water. Allow it to sit for a few minutes until it thickens into a gel-like consistency. Use this mixture as an egg substitute in recipes that call for eggs. It works well in muffins, cakes, cookies, and pancakes.

2. Enhancing Texture and Nutritional Value:

- Add a few tablespoons of chia seeds directly into your batter or dough. They can enhance the texture, providing a delightful crunch or pop, while also increasing the nutritional value of your baked goods.

3. Chia Flour:

- Grind chia seeds into a fine powder using a blender or food processor to create chia flour. You can replace a portion of regular flour in recipes with chia flour to boost the fiber, protein, and omega-3 content.

4. Moisture Retention:

- Chia seeds can help retain moisture in baked goods. Their

ability to absorb liquid can keep cakes, bread, or muffins moist for longer periods.

5. Seeding and Sprinkling:

- Sprinkle whole chia seeds on top of bread, rolls, or pastry dough before baking to add a decorative touch and a nutritious boost. It can also provide a delightful crunch to the finished product.

6. Adjusting Recipes:

- When adding chia seeds to baked goods, it's advisable to slightly increase the liquid content of the recipe as the seeds absorb moisture. Experiment with small adjustments until you achieve the desired consistency.

7. Chia Seed Puddings and Fillings:

- Use chia seed pudding or a thick chia gel as a filling for pastries, pies, or as a layer in cakes. The gel-like consistency can provide both flavor and texture to your baked creations.

Tips for Baking with Chia Seeds:

- **Proper Ratios:** When using chia gel as an egg substitute, maintain the ratio of 1 tablespoon of chia seeds to 3 tablespoons of water to replace one egg.

- **Experiment Gradually:** Start by adding small amounts of chia seeds to your recipes and gradually increase the quantity to understand how they affect texture and moisture.

Incorporating chia seeds into your baking endeavors, you can add nutritional value, texture, and unique characteristics to your baked goods while exploring their versatility in different recipes.

4.3 Chia Seeds in Beverages

Chia seeds can be a fantastic addition to various beverages, offering a nutritional boost, interesting textures, and versatility. Here's how you can incorporate chia seeds into your drinks:

1. Chia Seed Water:

Basic Chia Water:

- Add a tablespoon of chia seeds to a glass or bottle of water and let it sit for 10-15 minutes. Stir or shake the mixture

occasionally to prevent
clumping. You can flavor it
with a splash of lemon, lime, or
a natural sweetener like honey
or agave syrup.

Infused Chia Water:

- Create flavored chia water by
  infusing the water with your
  choice of fruits, herbs, or
  spices. Mix chia seeds into the
  infused water for a refreshing,
  nutrient-rich beverage.

2. Chia Seed Lemonade or Fruit Juices:

Chia Seed Lemonade:

- Mix chia seeds into freshly
  squeezed lemonade for added
  texture and a nutritional boost.
  The seeds absorb some of the

liquid, creating a slightly thicker consistency.

Chia Seed Fruit Juices:

- Stir chia seeds into fruit juices like orange juice or berry blends. Let the seeds soak for a few minutes to absorb some liquid and add texture to the juice.

3. Smoothies and Shakes:

Chia Seed Smoothies:

- Blend chia seeds directly into your smoothies for an extra nutritional punch. The seeds won't significantly alter the flavor but will add thickness and texture.

4. Chia Seed Teas and Coffees:

Chia Seed Tea:

- Mix chia seeds into herbal teas or green teas for a unique texture and added nutrients. Allow the seeds to soak in the warm tea to expand and form a gel-like consistency.

Chia Seed Coffee:

- Sprinkle chia seeds into your coffee and stir well. The seeds can add texture and a nutritional boost to your morning brew.

5. Chia Seed Milk:

Chia Seed Almond or Coconut Milk:

- Blend chia seeds with almond milk, coconut milk, or any other plant-based milk. Let the mixture sit for a while to thicken and create a chia-infused milk that can be used in various recipes or enjoyed on its own.

Tips for Chia Seed Beverages:

- **Soaking Time:** Allow chia seeds to soak for at least 10-15 minutes in liquids to achieve their gel-like texture and avoid clumping.

- **Stirring or Shaking:** Periodically stir or shake beverages containing chia seeds to prevent them from settling at the bottom.

CHAPTER 5

How to Buy and Store Chia Seeds

5.1 Selecting Quality Chia Seeds

When purchasing chia seeds, consider these tips to ensure you're getting high-quality seeds:

1. Look for Organic and Raw:

- Opt for organic chia seeds whenever possible to minimize exposure to pesticides and chemicals. Raw chia seeds retain their nutritional value better than processed varieties.

2. Check for Freshness and Smell:

- Inspect the seeds for freshness. They should have a mild, nutty aroma. Avoid chia seeds that smell rancid or musty, as this could indicate spoilage or improper storage.

3. Color and Texture:

- Quality chia seeds are typically uniform in color, ranging from black to white, and have a uniform size. Avoid seeds that appear discolored or have a dull appearance. They should also feel dry to the touch and not be clumped together.

4. Packaging and Brand Reputation:

- Purchase chia seeds from reputable brands or suppliers known for their quality. Ensure the seeds are packed in airtight containers or sealed bags to maintain freshness and prevent exposure to moisture.

5. Certification and Labels:

- Look for certifications such as USDA Organic, non-GMO, or any other quality assurance labels that indicate adherence to specific standards and quality control measures.

6. Read Reviews and Expiry Dates:

- Check reviews or ratings of the brand or product to gauge customer satisfaction and product quality. Additionally, pay attention to the expiry or "best by" date to ensure freshness.

Storage Recommendations for Chia Seeds:

1. Airtight Container:

- Transfer chia seeds into an airtight container or resealable bag once opened. Store them away from direct sunlight in a cool, dry place, like a pantry or cupboard.

2. Avoid Moisture:

- Keep chia seeds away from moisture and humidity, as exposure to moisture can cause them to spoil or clump together.

3. Proper Sealing:

- Ensure the container or bag is tightly sealed after each use to maintain the seeds' freshness and prevent them from absorbing moisture.

4. Shelf Life:

- Chia seeds have a relatively long shelf life, typically lasting up to two years when stored properly. However, for optimal freshness and nutritional value, it's best to use them within a reasonable timeframe.

Selecting high-quality chia seeds and storing them properly, you can ensure that they retain their nutritional value and freshness for an extended period, allowing you to enjoy their benefits in various culinary endeavors.

5.2 Proper Storage Techniques

Proper storage techniques are essential to maintaining the quality and freshness of chia seeds over time. Chia seeds, like many other seeds, can be sensitive to environmental factors such as light, heat, moisture, and air. By following appropriate storage practices, you can ensure that your chia seeds remain nutritious and flavorful for an extended period. Here's a detailed exploration of proper storage techniques for chia seeds:

1. **Container Selection:**

    - Choose an airtight container to store chia seeds. A glass or plastic container with a tight-sealing lid works well to keep out air and moisture. The container should be clean and dry before adding the chia seeds.

2. **Cool and Dark Location:**

    - Store the chia seeds in a cool, dark place.

Exposure to light and heat can accelerate the oxidation process and degrade the quality of the seeds. A pantry or cupboard away from direct sunlight and heat sources is an ideal location.

3. **Avoid Temperature Fluctuations:**

- Chia seeds are sensitive to temperature fluctuations. Avoid storing them in areas where temperatures vary significantly. Sudden temperature changes can lead to condensation inside the container, promoting mold growth

and reducing the shelf
life of the seeds.

4. **Refrigeration Option:**

- While chia seeds do not
  require refrigeration,
  storing them in the
  refrigerator can extend
  their freshness. If you
  live in a warm or humid
  climate, refrigerating
  chia seeds is a prudent
  choice. Ensure that the
  container is tightly sealed
  to prevent the seeds from
  absorbing moisture.

5. **Keep Away from Moisture:**

- Moisture is the enemy of
  chia seeds. Even a small
  amount of moisture can
  lead to clumping and
  spoilage. Store chia seeds

in a dry environment and avoid introducing wet utensils or scoops into the container. Consider adding a silica gel packet to absorb any residual moisture.

6. **Monitor Expiry Dates:**

   - Chia seeds have a relatively long shelf life, but it's crucial to monitor the expiration date on the packaging. Using chia seeds beyond their expiration date may result in a loss of nutritional value and freshness.

7. **Bulk Storage Considerations:**

   - If you purchase chia seeds in bulk, consider

dividing them into smaller portions for regular use. This minimizes the frequency of opening the main storage container, reducing exposure to air and moisture.

8. **Seal the Container Properly:**

- Before storing the chia seeds, make sure the container is sealed tightly after each use. This prevents air from entering and maintains the seeds' quality over time.

Adhering to these proper storage techniques, you can maximize the shelf life and preserve the nutritional integrity of chia seeds, ensuring that

they remain a versatile and healthful
addition to your diet.

CHAPTER 6

Potential Risks and Precautions

6.1 Allergies and Interactions

Chia seeds are generally considered safe for consumption, and they offer a range of health benefits. However, it's important to be aware of potential allergies and interactions that may arise, particularly for individuals with certain health conditions. Here's a detailed exploration of allergies and interactions associated with chia seeds:

1. **Allergies:**

- Chia seeds come from the Salvia hispanica plant and belong to the mint family. Individuals with known allergies to plants in the Lamiaceae family, such as mint, basil, and oregano, may be at an increased risk of chia seed allergies. Common allergic reactions include itching, swelling, hives, and, in severe cases, anaphylaxis. If you suspect an allergy, it is advisable to consult with a healthcare professional for proper evaluation.

2. **Cross-Allergenicity:**

- Cross-allergenicity is a phenomenon where individuals allergic to certain foods may also react to similar proteins in other foods. Although rare, individuals with allergies to mustard, sesame seeds, or other seeds may experience cross-allergenic reactions to chia seeds. If there is a known seed allergy, cautious introduction and monitoring of chia seed consumption are recommended.

3. **Gastrointestinal Sensitivity:**

- Chia seeds are high in fiber, and some individuals may experience gastrointestinal discomfort, such as bloating, gas, or abdominal cramps, especially when consuming large quantities or if not adequately hydrated. It is advisable to start with smaller amounts and gradually increase intake to allow the digestive system to adjust.

4. Medication Interactions:

- Chia seeds can absorb water and form a gel-like consistency. In some cases, this property may interfere with the absorption of certain medications. If you are taking medications, especially those for blood sugar regulation or blood-thinning, it's advisable to consult with a healthcare professional before incorporating large amounts of chia seeds into your diet.

5. Hydration:

- Due to their high fiber content, chia seeds can absorb a significant amount of water. It is crucial to consume chia seeds with an adequate amount of fluids to prevent the seeds from expanding in the digestive tract, which could potentially lead to choking or blockages. Individuals with difficulty swallowing or a history of esophageal issues should exercise caution when consuming chia seeds.

6.2 Usage Caution

While chia seeds are celebrated for their nutritional value and versatility, it is essential to exercise caution in their usage to ensure a safe and enjoyable culinary experience. Here are specific precautions and considerations to keep in mind when incorporating chia seeds into your diet:

1. **Hydration is Key:**

    - Chia seeds have the unique ability to absorb large amounts of liquid and form a gel-like consistency. To prevent potential issues, such as choking or digestive discomfort, it's crucial to hydrate chia seeds adequately before consuming them. Soaking them in water or other liquids for at least 15 minutes or until they achieve a gel-like texture is advisable.

2. **Moderation in Consumption:**

- While chia seeds offer various health benefits, moderation is key. Excessive consumption may lead to an increased intake of fiber, which, in some cases, could cause gastrointestinal discomfort, bloating, or gas. Start with small amounts and gradually

increase as your
digestive system adapts.

3. **Individual Tolerance:**

   - Every individual's tolerance to new foods can vary. Some people may be more sensitive to the introduction of high-fiber foods like chia seeds. Pay attention to how your body responds and adjust your intake accordingly. If you experience any adverse reactions, consult with a healthcare professional.

4. **Nutrient Diversity:**

   - While chia seeds are nutrient-dense, they should be part of a well-balanced diet. Relying solely on chia seeds for specific nutrients may lead to an imbalance in your overall nutrient intake. Incorporate a variety of foods to ensure a diverse and comprehensive nutritional profile.

5. **Pre-existing Medical Conditions:**

- Individuals with certain medical conditions, such as swallowing difficulties, gastrointestinal disorders, or a history of bowel obstructions, should exercise caution when consuming chia seeds. Consult with a healthcare professional to determine

if chia seeds are suitable
for your specific health
situation.

6. **Allergies and Sensitivities:**

- Be aware of potential
  allergies or sensitivities
  to chia seeds, especially
  if you have a history of
  allergies to seeds or other
  related foods. Monitor
  for any allergic reactions,
  and seek medical
  attention if symptoms
  occur.

7. **Quality of Chia Seeds:**

- Ensure that the chia
  seeds you purchase are of
  high quality. Purchase
  from reputable sources to
  minimize the risk of
  contamination. Check for

any signs of spoilage, such as an off odor or mold, before consumption.

8. **Child and Pet Safety:**

    - Chia seeds, when hydrated, can form a gel-like substance. Keep hydrated chia seeds away from small children to prevent the risk of choking. Additionally, be cautious with pets, as some may be attracted to the texture and smell of chia seeds.

9. **Consultation with Healthcare Professionals:**

    - If you have any pre-existing health conditions, are pregnant,

or are taking
medications, it's
advisable to consult with
a healthcare professional
before introducing chia
seeds into your diet.
They can provide
personalized advice
based on your individual
health status.

Incorporating chia seeds mindfully
and being aware of these usage
cautions, you can enjoy the nutritional
benefits of chia seeds while
minimizing the risk of potential
complications. Listen to your body,
practice moderation, and seek
professional guidance if needed.

6.3 Myth Busting

Chia seeds have gained popularity for their nutritional benefits, but like many foods, they are not immune to misconceptions. Let's debunk some common myths associated with chia seeds:

1. **Myth: Chia Seeds Expand in Your Body and Can Cause Blockages.**

    - *Reality:* Chia seeds do absorb water and expand, but the idea that they can cause blockages in your digestive system is a myth. When consumed with sufficient fluids, chia seeds form a gel-like substance in the stomach, aiding digestion and promoting a feeling of fullness.

2. **Myth: Chia Seeds Can Replace Meals for Weight Loss.**

- *Reality:* While chia seeds are nutrient-dense and can be part of a weight-loss plan, they should not be relied upon as a meal replacement. A balanced diet with a variety of foods is essential for overall health. Chia seeds can contribute to a feeling of fullness, but they should be part of a well-rounded diet.

3. **Myth: Chia Seeds Contain Too Many Calories for a Healthy Diet.**

- *Reality:* Chia seeds are indeed calorie-dense due

to their healthy fat content. However, they provide valuable nutrients like omega-3 fatty acids, fiber, and protein. When consumed in moderation as part of a balanced diet, the nutritional benefits of chia seeds outweigh their calorie content.

4. **Myth: Chia Seeds Can Cure All Health Ailments.**

- *Reality:* While chia seeds offer numerous health benefits, they are not a cure-all. Claims that they can treat specific diseases or replace medical treatments are unfounded. Chia seeds should be seen as a supportive element in a healthy lifestyle rather than a sole solution for health issues.

5. **Myth: Only Soaking Chia Seeds Overnight Makes Them Safe to Eat.**

   - *Reality:* While soaking chia seeds can enhance their digestibility, it is not the only way to consume them safely. Chia seeds can also be sprinkled on top of foods or added to recipes without soaking. The key is to ensure adequate fluid intake, whether from soaking or consuming them with liquids.

6. **Myth: Chia Seeds Are High in Omega-3 Fatty Acids Like Fish.**

   - *Reality:* While chia seeds do contain omega-3 fatty acids, they provide a different type called alpha-linolenic acid (ALA), not the same as the omega-3s found in fish. While ALA is beneficial, it may not have the same heart health benefits as the EPA and DHA found in fatty fish.

7. **Myth: Chia Seeds Are Only for Vegans and Vegetarians.**

   - *Reality:* Chia seeds are a versatile food suitable for a variety of dietary preferences. While they are an excellent plant-based source of protein and omega-3 fatty acids, they can be enjoyed by individuals with different dietary patterns, including omnivores.

8. **Myth: Chia Seeds Expire Quickly.**

   - *Reality:* Chia seeds have a relatively long shelf life when stored properly. While they can go rancid over time, following appropriate storage techniques, such as keeping them in a cool, dark place in an airtight container, can extend their freshness.

By dispelling these myths, we can better appreciate chia seeds for what they are—a nutritious and versatile addition to a balanced diet. It's crucial to base our understanding of food on scientific evidence and maintain a realistic perspective on their benefits.

6.4 Embracing Chia Seeds in Daily Life

Chia seeds are a nutritional powerhouse that can be easily incorporated into your daily routine, enhancing both the flavor and health benefits of your meals. Here are some creative and practical ways to embrace chia seeds in your daily life:

1. **Chia Pudding Breakfast:**

   - Start your day with a nutritious chia pudding.

Mix chia seeds with your favorite plant-based milk (such as almond or coconut) and let it sit in the refrigerator overnight. Top it with fresh fruits, nuts, and a drizzle of honey for a delicious and satisfying breakfast.

2. **Smoothie Boost:**

- Add a tablespoon of chia seeds to your morning smoothie for an extra boost of fiber, protein, and omega-3 fatty acids. The seeds will add a subtle crunch and contribute to the overall thickness of your smoothie.

3. **Salad Topper:**

- Sprinkle chia seeds on top of salads to enhance their nutritional profile. The seeds add a mild, nutty flavor and a delightful crunch. They pair well with a variety of greens, vegetables, and protein sources.

4. **Baking and Cooking:**

- Incorporate chia seeds into your baking recipes. They can be added to muffins, pancakes, and bread for a nutritional twist. Chia seeds can also serve as an egg substitute in recipes, making them suitable for vegan baking.

5. **Yogurt Parfait:**

- Create a wholesome yogurt parfait by layering Greek yogurt, chia seeds, granola, and fresh berries. This makes for a satisfying and nutrient-rich snack or dessert option.

6. **Hydrating Chia Water:**

- Infuse your water with chia seeds for a hydrating and refreshing drink. Mix chia seeds with water, a splash of lemon or lime juice, and a touch of natural sweetener. Allow it to sit for a few minutes, and enjoy a naturally flavored chia-infused beverage.

7. **Chia Seed Jam:**

- Make your own
  nutritious jam by
  combining chia seeds
  with mashed berries and
  a sweetener of your
  choice. This homemade
  jam is a healthier
  alternative to store-
  bought versions, and it's
  simple to prepare.

8. **Trail Mix Upgrade:**

- Enhance your favorite
  trail mix by including
  chia seeds. Combine
  them with nuts, dried
  fruits, and dark chocolate
  for a satisfying and
  energy-boosting snack.

9. **Chia Seed Oatmeal:**

- Stir chia seeds into your morning oatmeal for added texture and nutritional benefits. Top it with sliced bananas, nuts, and a sprinkle of cinnamon for a hearty and wholesome breakfast.

10. **Chia Seed Energy Bars:**

- Make your own energy bars by mixing chia seeds with ingredients like oats, nut butter, and honey. Press the mixture into a pan, refrigerate, and cut into bars for a convenient and nutritious snack.

11. **Chia Seed Dressings:**

- Create homemade salad
  dressings by blending
  chia seeds with olive oil,
  vinegar, and your
  favorite herbs and spices.
  This not only adds a
  nutritional boost but also
  contributes to the creamy
  texture of the dressing.

By incorporating chia seeds into your
daily meals and snacks, you can enjoy
their nutritional benefits in a variety
of delicious and creative ways.
Experiment with different recipes to
find the perfect fit for your taste
preferences and dietary needs.